Sleep

While You're Still Alive

Good

News

from a

Former

Insomniac

Audrey Wagner

ISBN: 1545300356
ISBN-13: 978-1545300350

CONTENTS

1 WHAT IT'S ABOUT

I don't know where you are on the "I can't sleep" continuum. Your sleep may be mediocre, or it may be almost nonexistent. Maybe life stressors and aging have taken a toll on your sleep. Or you got insomnia abruptly and can't seem to get back on track. However poor your sleep is, I know your suffering (more on that in the next chapter).

I wrote this book because I have something special to offer you. Conventional sleep tips were not enough to help me sleep. A heavy tranquilizer nearly destroyed my life. But I was shocked when a unique combination of foods and nutrients cured my insomnia. I've slept well for almost ten years now because of them. I am going to share them with you.

I've done rigorous research for this book, but I'll present it to you in as few words as possible. After all, you're eager to get back to sleep at night. And you want to get started with simple, concrete actions.

Beginning in Chapter 7, that's what I'll give you. Until then, I'm going to explain how I got there and why my recommendations make sense.

2 I'M A FORMER INSOMNIAC

My first job out of graduate school was...stressful. I hadn't been a good sleeper during my graduate school years, then job stress took this problem to a new level. After a few weeks of unmanageable stress, I went five straight days without sleep (yes, I know that's hard to believe). My local doctor wrote me a prescription for a large dose of Klonopin—a tranquilizer in a category of drugs called benzodiazepines. I later learned that the amount he prescribed me was enough to knock out a grizzly bear or an adolescent moose. My point is, he started me off on a very heavy dose.

The night I filled that prescription was the beginning of a very dark period. To call it a nightmare would be a compliment. You can read my full story in my memoir *Klonopin Withdrawal and Howling Dogs*, available on Amazon.

What is important for you to know is, when it comes to insomnia, *I've been there.* I've gone days without sleep. I've felt like a zombie and desperately wanted out of my skin. I've been misjudged by people who think insomnia just points to psychological problems. I've wished for a brain transplant (do they have those?). After I weaned off Klonopin, the withdrawal insomnia was so horrific that I thought about death around the clock for two and a half months straight and wondered if I would *ever sleep again.*

Fast-forward to now. This fall marks ten years since my recovery from insomnia. In the years since my recovery, I have slept well. I rarely have insomnia, and when I do, it's only because I'm not following my own recommendations in this book! When I follow them, I sleep great. In fact, I sleep better now as an adult in my late 30s than I did in my 20s before my sleep problems got really bad.

Now you're wondering how I got from point A to point B. I will tell you exactly how later in this book. But, the first thing I had to do was get off—and stay off—sleeping pills.

3 GO TO THE DOCTOR?

Insomnia, the most common sleep disorder, is difficulty falling or staying asleep or poor quality sleep that results in some level of daytime impairment.[i] Insomnia affects about 33-50% of the population, though those meeting the diagnostic criteria (reporting distress or daytime impairment) are 10-15% of the population.[ii]

In the words of Dr. Abigail Zuger, insomnia is being "medicalized."[iii] We are told by popular healthcare sites, like The National Sleep Foundation and Mayo Clinic, to contact our doctors for insomnia. [iv][v] They and the National Institute of Health say insomnia is "treated" with cognitive and behavioral changes or prescription sleeping pills.[vi]

But insomnia is not an illness or a disease. Even our healthcare system admits it is *just a symptom*.[vii] Mayo Clinic says it usually results from "stress, life events or habits that disrupt sleep," also saying it may be associated with a medical condition, drugs, or aging.[viii] Even sleep doctor Dr. Tom Scammel admits that most insomniacs don't have anything wrong with their ability to sleep but rather with their poor habits—the things they are eating and drinking, and too much mental stimulation at night.[ix]

It is alarming that our healthcare system is medicalizing insomnia, while at the same time admitting it's not a medical problem!

Even worse, sleeping pills are harmful. The American Academy of Sleep Medicine (AASM) published a clinical guideline in 2017 with their conclusion about sleeping pills (hint—it's grim). Their verdict is.... (get ready for it)... commonly prescribed sleeping pills are *not recommended*.[x]

This is why. Studies on sleeping pills provide low quality evidence. First of all, the data is inconsistent. Secondly, the studies are funded by the companies selling the drugs! Lastly, the negative effects of sleeping pills are not included in the studies.[xi] Yikes.

But the negative effects are real, and the AASM lists them.[xii] Also, Dr. Daniel Kripke published his comprehensive review showing sleeping pills cause excess mortality, infections, increased cancer, clinical depression, accidents, withdrawal insomnia, and other withdrawal symptoms including anxiety, panic, and epilepsy.[xiii]

There's more bad news. The AASM admits that the benefits of sleeping pills stop as soon as you stop taking them.[xiv] Read: sleeping pills don't cure insomnia.

So, what are sleeping pills good for? Do they have benefits? Let's use a popular one, Ambien, for an example. The trials reviewed by the AASM found that Ambien increased sleep time by an average of 29 minutes.[xv] Dr. Kripke found that Z-drugs like Ambien and Imovane only increased sleep time by an average of 11 minutes in the studies he reviewed.[xvi]

In spite of these depressing facts, sleeping pills are "by far, the most common approach" to "treating" insomnia.[xvii] Doctors often prescribe them because they are not aware of non-drug approaches.[xviii] [xix]

The most ironic risk is that sleeping pills make insomnia worse. You read that right. Dr. Kripke states, "Randomized placebo-controlled clinical trials have now demonstrated that hypnotics do indeed cause insomnia." He reviewed trials involving commonly prescribed sleeping pills and found that people who take them ultimately end up with *more* insomnia.

But what about cognitive behavioral therapy? This includes things like using the bed only for sleep, limiting sleep time, relaxation exercises, changing unhelpful beliefs about sleep, and biofeedback.[xx] Two meta-analyses found this type of therapy only increased sleep time by averages of 17 minutes[xxi] and 7.61 minutes.[xxii] That doesn't sound like a whole lot more sleep to me.

It turns out that neither sleeping pills *nor* cognitive behavioral therapy are effectively solving people's sleep problems.[xxiii] Yet these are the foremost "treatment" options in our Western healthcare system!

So, should you go to the doctor for insomnia, as conventional advice tells you to? If you have a medical condition or a sleep disorder that requires medical attention, the doctor can help. But if you *just can't sleep...* then read on. See what the research has to say about the true causes of insomnia and the exciting cure they all share.

4 IF YOU "JUST CAN'T SLEEP"

If you have insomnia, you might be wracking your brain, wondering what's wrong with you. I've been there. During my insomnia nightmare, I was very paranoid. Did I have heavy metal poisoning? Was something wrong with my brain? Did I have a disease that hadn't yet been discovered? Did I have deeply rooted psychological problems that were beyond help? I was simply dying to know the "cause" of my insomnia.

After I recovered from Klonopin withdrawal, I learned that the "cause" of my insomnia (other than sleeping pills, of course) had been nothing out of the ordinary. The cause of your insomnia probably isn't out of the ordinary either. To show you what I mean, we are going to look at inflammation, stress, caffeine, and aging in this chapter. These topics aren't as boring as they sound—you'll see why.

Inflammation

It turns out that pretty much all health problems are linked to chronic inflammation.[xxiv] Why should you care about inflammation? For the reason that matters to you: it's linked with insomnia! [xxv xxvi xxvii xxviii xxix] Chronic inflammation results from eating the unhealthy, nutrient-starved standard American diet.[xxx] [xxxi] Let's connect the dots: chronic inflammation is ultimately linked to *not having enough nutrients*. This conclusion is proven. Scientific studies have found that insomnia is associated with a lower nutrient intake[xxxii] and an unhealthy diet.[xxxiii]

Insomnia is also linked to stress, caffeine, and aging. Let's talk about these in order.

Stress

The authors of a fascinating *Sleep Medicine Clinics* journal show that insomnia is *really* about hyperarousal (stress) around the clock, and losing sleep is just one symptom of that.

In other words, insomniacs tend to be more stressed out.

Citing many studies, the authors found insomnia is connected to the following:[xxxiv]

- Stressful life events
- Being female (hormonal changes mean increased sensitivity to stress)
- Aging (increased sensitivity to stress)
- Being separated, divorced, or widowed
- Lower educational status
- Lower economic status
- Unemployment
- Discontentment
- Less satisfying personal relationships
- Poor self-concept

- Inadequate coping mechanisms for dealing with stress

- Depressed mood

- Rumination

- Chronic anxiety

- Inhibition of emotions

- Inability to express anger

- Mood and anxiety disorders

- Substance abuse disorders

- Certain medical conditions

- Smoking

- Alcohol

- Some prescription drugs

- Sleeping pill withdrawal

Note the number of things on that list that are directly or indirectly about stress!

Stress hormones can keep you in a state of arousal around the clock. But there's another downside to stress: it uses up and eliminates vitamins and minerals that you need to sleep well![xxxv] To make this worse, people under stress often eat more junk food, so their nutrient levels decrease even more. "I'm super stressed, so I'm just going to swing by the gas station and get one of those chocolate pies that come in a wrapper." (Shameful confession: I've eaten a few of those.)

Caffeine

We often use caffeine even more when we're stressed (it helps wash down the junk food). But scientific studies have found that caffeine causes insomnia.[xxxvi] [xxxvii] Not only that, but it also prevents the absorption of some nutrients that we really need for sleep![xxxviii] I love coffee as much as anyone, so I understand if you want to throw this book across the room. But I hope you don't, because the exciting conclusion of this chapter is yet to come.

Aging

Aging comes into the picture here. Older adults may be more sensitive to caffeine.[xxxix] People over 35 cannot tolerate the same level of caffeine as they could in their 20s and early 30s.[xl] I totally resonate. After I hit age 38, I had to cut my coffee down to *one cup or less* in the morning in order to sleep well at night! Yet another significant effect of aging is a decreased ability to absorb nutrients![xli]

Putting It All Together

You probably noticed a theme in this chapter that has something to do with not getting enough nutrients (if so, you nailed it). Insomnia is linked to poor diet, stress, caffeine, and aging. And each of these things results in insufficient nutrients. What this means is that insomnia is linked to *not getting enough nutrients*. Imagine that last sentence being blared from a megaphone next to your ear.

Are you eating like an American? Are you stressed, drinking caffeine, and aging? If you are any or all of these things, then you probably don't have enough nutrients in your body to sleep well—at least not until you make some changes. If you are a highly sensitive person like me, then insufficient nutrients could have a worse-than-average effect on you, as it does for me.

The good news is, all these links share a common cure, which is—you guessed it—*getting more nutrients!* This is the exciting conclusion I told you was coming, and I can only dream that you're as excited as I am.

The bottom line is that getting more nutrients helps people sleep better. More on that in the next chapter.

5 FOOD CAN PUT YOU TO SLEEP OR KEEP YOU AWAKE

Food can put you to sleep, or food can keep you awake.

I made the shocking discovery, after I recovered from Klonopin withdrawal, that my body is a natural sleeping pill. When I get the right things into it, *I sleep well at night!* Prescription tranquilizers don't hold a candle to the natural sleeping pill that my body becomes when I get certain foods and nutrients. Food has pretty much *everything* to do with my body becoming that natural sleeping pill.

You see, the standard American diet (also known as the Western diet) is a *triple whammy* when it comes to sleep. First, the food additives in processed foods excite the nervous system and keep you awake. Second, the Western diet doesn't have enough nutrients to put you to sleep. Third, the Western diet can give you diseases that make it difficult to sleep.

I know it's really hard to believe that food is more powerful than drugs in giving you a good night's sleep. But it is! You might be feeling skeptical when I say that. So I'll show you.

We saw in the previous chapter that studies show insomnia is linked to a lower nutrient intake and an unhealthy diet. Even more studies reveal that nutrients have a lot to do with sleep. For example, people sleep better with more magnesium and zinc.[xlii] Sleep is improved by potassium, calcium, magnesium, iron, zinc, vitamin A, vitamin D, thiamin, riboflavin, vitamin B6, and folate, as well as certain food groups, including vegetables.[xliii] Deficiencies in selenium and Vitamin C are linked to poor sleep, and better sleep is linked to getting calcium, Vitamin D, lycopene, and potassium.[xliv] Potassium[xlv] and magnesium[xlvi] [xlvii] in the diet led to better sleep. Even kiwifruit has specifically been found to improve sleep. [xlviii] We'll touch on more related studies in chapters to come.

It make sense, really. Dr. Arden Anderson explains that just as a computer is correlated to its software and hardware, the functions of the body are correlated to nutrition.[xlix] This includes the body processes that make us fall asleep!

I remember going to the Walmart pharmacy and purchasing my first over the counter sleep aid (before I got prescribed Klonopin). I was totally clueless back in those days—I had no idea that food had *anything* to do with sleep. I wouldn't discover that until after my recovery from Klonopin withdrawal. When that time came, I was shocked that nutrients were working to put me to sleep.

That's what the rest of my book is about. I'm going to tell you *exactly* what I do to sleep well every night. But before I can tell you, I have one more important thing to say...

6 DON'T FEED THESE TO THE BIRDS

No matter how many nutrients you take in, you could still get insomnia if you're sleeping until noon, getting into bed too early, drinking too much coffee, sleeping with your iPhone, or wearing tight jeans to bed.

You might be a serious insomniac, like I was. You might think sleep tips can't be taken seriously, that they're for people who fall asleep with lavender under their pillows. When I was in the throes of insomnia, I figured that common sleep tips should be fed to the birds. But, although insomnia can make us feel crazy, it really can be caused by simple things such as being in front of the television at night.

Dr. Mercola can give you pretty much *all* great sleep tips in his article, "Top 33 Tips to Optimize Your Sleep Routine."[1] I encourage you to check them out.

I'll tell you which ones I personally *must* do for a good night's sleep. Not even my own recommendations would work for me if I didn't follow these basic sleep tips!

- I stick to a regular sleeping schedule and never go to bed early. I find that 10:30 p.m. to 6:30 a.m., or 11 to 7, is a good schedule for me. On weekend nights I sometimes sleep 11:30 to 7:30. Sometimes I sleep in Saturday mornings, but not often.

- I sleep in a cool room, 69 degrees or cooler.

- I sleep with a sound machine.

- I also sleep with earplugs (I like muffled white noise. It may sound strange, but it keeps me from being woken up by thunder, people talking, dogs barking, etc.).

- I sleep with loose, soft clothing (anything tight or uncomfortable can distract from sleep).

- I abstain from heavy exercise at least three hours before bed. I can get away with an evening walk a couple of hours before bedtime. But my heartrate needs to be totally slowed down before I can fall asleep.

- I abstain from hot baths or showers at least three hours before bed. (Hot baths are great for sleep when taken earlier in the day or evening, but taking them too late at night keeps my body from cooling down). If I take a late night shower, I make sure it's cool to lukewarm. If you have the nerve, cold showers and baths right before bed are supposed to knock you out cold (pun intended).

- Alcohol and caffeine are no-no's for me. I usually have one 8-oz cup of coffee (or less) in the mornings. And I usually avoid alcohol, especially in the evenings.

- I get away from cell phones, televisions, and computers by 9 p.m. That way, by 10:30 p.m., I'm able to fall asleep. Looking at electronics after 9 p.m. never fails to postpone my ability to fall asleep.

- I don't go to bed hungry, and I don't under-eat in general. I get that we need a calorie deficit in order to lose weight. But my calorie deficit can't be large, or else I can't sleep. Generally, undereating causes insomnia.[li] If you want to have a calorie deficit, make sure yours isn't severe enough to disrupt your sleep.

I believe common sleep tips are crucial. Although they aren't sufficient to put me to sleep, they're necessary. With sleep tips in tow, I'm ready to tell you what *is* sufficient to put me to sleep every night.

But the first one is about something I *don't* do.

7 STOP EATING FRANKENFOODS

Remember that insomnia is linked to poor diet. To start getting some much needed sleep, eat real food. This means you should generally avoid the modern Western diet. You know those boxed and canned foods with loooooong lists of ingredients you don't recognize? Don't eat those.

I'm not telling you to go on any particular diet. Dr. Weston A. Price discovered that traditional diets had a lot of variety. People ate high fat, low fat, high carb, meat only, plants only, milk, blood, blubber, or any whole food you can imagine.[lii] My point is, I believe you can sleep well eating a lot of different diets—as long as it's not the Western one.

So...what is the Western diet? It's a diet with lots of "Frankenfoods"—processed junk foods and fast foods. Right now, the food additives list on the FDA site has 3,971 items![liii]

There are even more things wrong with the Western diet. I'm sure you've heard of factory farms—where animals raised in feedlots aren't healthy. The meat and dairy from these animals isn't ideal. I'm sure you've heard of pesticides, too—chemicals used to grow produce. And you've probably seen warnings in the media about how we eat way too much white flour and white sugar. Also, those cheap vegetable oils are bad news.

But who wants to waste time learning all about the unhealthy Western diet? Better to just kick it to the curb.

You may not be ready to live off the grid and raise all of your own food. You may not be able to afford raw cream and grass-fed beef from a nearby farm. Maybe buying all organic produce would hurt your bank account. I totally get that. I do not perfectly avoid the Western diet. Sometimes I don't know what's in the food I'm eating at other people's houses and at restaurants. Sometimes I buy some produce that's not organic and cheese that wasn't made from grass-fed animals.

However, there are foods I avoid *with a ten-foot pole.* And I'm telling you about them so you can avoid them, too, and then you'll have a prayer for sleep.

The first is vegetable oils. Modern vegetable oils, mostly from soy, corn, safflower and canola, are processed with high heat and solvents; they increase inflammation.[liv] (Remember, inflammation is linked to insomnia). Margarine and vegetable shortening are even worse due to their chemical changes.[lv]

Safe oils that are easily accessible include avocado oil, high quality olive oil, and coconut oil.

The second group of "foods" to avoid are artificial sweeteners and MSG. These are also called "excitotoxins." They don't help you get to dream-land.

Of the 3,971 food additives in America, excitotoxins are not the *only* harmful ones. But I focus on them because these not-so-exciting excitotoxins excite the nervous system. Insomniacs should run from them. There are many names for artificial sweeteners and MSG . What they all have in common is they can keep you awake.[lvi] [lvii]

The best study is the one you can do on yourself: avoid MSG and artificial sweeteners. Do a current search for the many names of artificial sweeteners and MSG, because new ones could be added. Then check your chewing gum, mints, candy, and beverages, along with your foods.

By eliminating foods with vegetable oils and long lists of unrecognizable ingredients (but especially excitotoxins), you automatically cut out fast food and junk food and, therefore, eliminate the majority of Frankenfoods from your diet. Just like magic.

I avoid almost all food additives. I even have to avoid a common ingredient called "natural flavors." Do flavors grow on trees or in the ground? They don't. My nervous system doesn't like them.

If you want more information about eating an anti-inflammatory diet, Dr. Steven Gundry (gundrymd.com), Dr. Joseph Mercola (mercola.com), and the Weston A. Price Foundation (westonaprice.org), have lots of great information.

But I've got *much* more exciting information for you...

After kicking inflammatory foods to the curb, you can give yourself some specific foods and nutrients that will *really* knock you out. They are... sleep powerhouses. Or should I say sleep bombs? I don't know. But they are the fastest nutritional trains to dreamland. They will help you sleep while you're still alive.

Before you learn them, an analogy will help.

Think of a car that isn't running. A car mechanic spends the day trying to find out what is wrong. He can't figure it out, so he replaces some expensive parts hoping that will make the car run. At the end of a long, exhausting day, he still can't get the car to move. He then sees that the car has no fuel!

The nutritional actions in the next chapters are intimately tied to body processes that promote sleep. Other natural insomnia cures may not work if you're not getting the right stuff into your body to begin with—just as repairs won't help the car run if the car's out of fuel.

But if you *do* get the right stuff into your body, then sleep tips could start working for you. Other foods and nutrients that are not in this book could help, too.

Since the following recommendations are foundational for a good night's sleep, I hope they will become a part of your daily life.

Let's see what they are.

8 DRINK THESE EVERY DAY

All foods can be healthy in their natural states. But this doesn't mean that no foods are special. When it comes to sleep, it turns out that some foods are *very* special.

Victoria Boutenko did rigorous research and learned that greens are the food that best matches all human nutritional needs.[lviii]

Don't throw this book across the room (again). This chapter isn't about making mustard greens on the stove every night. I promise. So let's keep going.

Greens contain at least some of *each* essential vitamin and mineral, where data was available.[lix] Dang... greens are pretty awesome.

Boutenko studied cellulose, the primary building block of green plants. The nutrients are stored inside this tough material, and only when the cell walls are ruptured can nutrients be released. Our jaws are too weak to chew greens enough to rupture their cell walls. So, the simple way to "rupture" the cellulose, releasing their nutrients, is with a blender![lx] Thank goodness for technology.

It turns out that greens smoothies will really help you sleep. Boutenko and her family provided green smoothies for 27 volunteers who agreed to drink one quart of green smoothie per day for a month. In the post-study questionnaires, 19 of the 27 participants reported sleeping better—some of them *much* better![lxi] And improving sleep wasn't even the goal of the study!

But it's not surprising that the volunteers slept better. Of all foods, organic greens are among the highest in the sleep-inducing nutrients magnesium, calcium, and potassium. Those nutrients help us sleep better.[lxii] Sleep suffers for people who have deficiencies in calcium[lxiii] [lxiv] and magnesium.[lxv] [lxvi]

Spinach and Swiss Chard are where it's at. Dr. Mercola recommends them for their levels of magnesium and potassium.[lxvii] Spinach and Swiss chard are succeeded only by pumpkin seeds in foods with the most magnesium.[lxviii] Spinach and Swiss chard rank third and ninth in foods with the most calcium, both beating kale.[lxix] Lastly, Swiss chard and spinach rate second and third on the list of foods with the most potassium.[lxx] (The World's Healthiest Foods website only includes commonly accessible greens. However, Boutenko's list of greens also includes wild edible weeds as well as root vegetable tops, herbs, and sprouts).[lxxi]

Because they are the commonly available greens highest in magnesium, calcium and potassium, I consider spinach and Swiss chard fantastic for green smoothies. Spinach is my green of choice for smoothies, as it has a little more calcium than Swiss chard and is commonly available organic in large plastic tubs you can put right into the freezer.

Green smoothies are my number one sleep cure. I recommend drinking at least one green smoothie every day. To make one, put at least two large handfuls of organic spinach or Swiss chard (or other dark, leafy greens) into a high-powered blender with some liquid. Blend and drink. You can simply add water to your greens and blend for the simplest green smoothie ever made, which I call "the lazy person's green smoothie." Maybe no one else has been this lazy, because I can't find this recipe on the internet.

Fortunately for you, there are endless delicious green smoothie recipes on the web. Regardless of the recipe, don't go light on the greens—I recommend at least a couple large handfuls. Also, throw at least a little fat in (a few nuts or seeds, etc.), because some nutrients require fat to be absorbed.[lxxii]

Right now you may be wondering if you can just take calcium, magnesium, and potassium as supplements instead of drinking green smoothies.

The answer is no...

I can't *believe* you were looking for a shortcut! ;-)

I have taken magnesium and calcium supplements many times for extra mineral support. However, I noticed that taking those did not help me sleep if I did not also drink green smoothies. Nutrients are delivered to us more effectively when they come from food because food contains "hundreds of carotenoids, flavonoids, minerals, and antioxidants," according to Dr. Clifford Lo.[lxxiii] Likewise, our bodies can't absorb supplements properly unless we are getting enough nutrition from food."[lxxiv]

I can totally see why you want to get out of drinking something green. But I don't believe there are any shortcuts. I have tried many times to sleep without green smoothies, but my sleep suffered every time. (Dang it.)

Green smoothies truly knock me out. I even travel with a blender and greens. Try them, and you'll sleep while you're still alive.

9 DON'T UNDERESTIMATE THESE

Wouldn't it be great if we could get enough nutrients from what we are eating? Theoretically, we could...

Except for a few unfortunate facts about our modern lifestyles:

1. We don't eat enough nutritious food.
2. Produce has less nutrients than it used to.

3. Stress, caffeine, and aging deplete our nutrients.

4. Our toxic environments deplete our nutrients.

Sadly, harvested food has declined in nutrients."[lxxv] [lxxvi] And our bodies are under assault from pollution, chemicals, and toxins that include pesticides, preservatives, artificial ingredients, antibiotics, hormones, and chemicals.[lxxvii] The Organic Consumers Association calls our exposure a "toxic soup of 100,000 synthetic chemicals that surround us every day."[lxxviii] Therefore, our need for nutrients is at an all-time high.

Even if we are eating healthy and drinking green smoothies every day, modern circumstances make getting enough nutrients challenging. So I think we should take multivitamins every day.

Multivitamins are recommended by many doctors and nutrition experts, but they've gotten a bad reputation. Some research says that multivitamins don't help or even cause cancer.

But these studies were about *synthetic* vitamins.[lxxix] Most synthetic vitamins are made from petroleum extracts, coal tar derivatives, and chemically processed sugars.[lxxx] Synthetic vitamins have a different structure, explains

Dr. Theil.[lxxxi] He cites a lot of research showing that synthetics don't have the same positive effects as food vitamins.[lxxxii]

Most *food* vitamins are made from acerola cherries, broccoli, cabbage, carrots, lemons, limes, nutritional yeast, oranges, and rice bran.[lxxxiii] That sounds quite sleep-inducing. (And a lot more appetizing than petroleum.)

You would be hard-pressed to find a 100% food multivitamin even in a vitamin store. Supplements that say "whole food," "grown in food," or "food-based" just mean they *contain* food along with synthetics. Such claims mislead people without technically lying.

In contrast, nutrients that are entirely food say "100% natural" or "100% food." Dr. Theil's Food Research, Inc. makes 100% natural whole food supplements that you can trust. Their many whole food supplements can be found at buyfoodresearch.com.

I took multivitamins with synthetics for years (and they helped me sleep, I admit) but I now take Dr. Thiel's 100% natural whole food supplements. Every day, I take his multivitamin called "Vitamin-Mineral" as well as his one called, "B-6, B-12 & folate" to get plenty of those stress-relieving B-vitamins! I feel as good and sleep as well as ever!

Remember, from Chapter 5, all the vitamins

and minerals shown by studies to help people sleep? Getting a wide array of nutrients through the extra support of multivitamins will help you sleep while you're still alive.

10 GET SUNSHINE INTO YOUR BODY

You probably remember how deeply you slept when you were a kid, after spending all day in the hot summer sun.

But we often don't get enough sunlight because of sunscreen, indoor jobs, and grey skies.[lxxxiv] Dr. Michael Holick says, "if you live above Atlanta, Georgia, you basically cannot make any vitamin D in your skin from about November through March."[lxxxv]

Yikes.

Vitamin D is hard to get from food unless you really, *really* like fish.[lxxxvi] (I don't... they're slimy and they swim). The Weston A. Price Foundation recommends supplementing with cod liver oil as a way to get more vitamin D[lxxxvii], but that can be expensive for many of us.

Vitamin D deficiency has negative effects on sleep.[lxxxviii] [lxxxix] So, unless you frequently sunbathe all year round somewhere below Atlanta, taking vitamin D3 is super important for your sleep. Supplemental vitamin D3 (cholecalciferol) may not be food-based, but it is sunshine-based— derived from the lanolin of sheep wool. That's natural enough for me!

But how much should you take? Sadly, the official recommendation of the U.S. government is way too low due to a mathematical error.[xc] And vitamin D deficiency is rampant[xci] and a public health problem.[xcii]

So you need to take a whole lot more than the official U.S. recommendation. The Vitamin D Council recommends 5,000 IU of vitamin D per day for adults, with 10,000 IU being the safe upper limit.[xciii] The way to know your exact D levels and needed dose is to get tested, which you can do through an in-home test kit.[xciv]

Although I haven't been tested, I won't say you shouldn't be.

I take 5,000 to 15,000 IU of vitamin D3 every morning (depending on the season). When I've gone without taking the sunshine vitamin (especially in the winter time!) my sleep has suffered. I take it in the mornings (taking it at night has hurt my sleep cycle).

The sunshine vitamin will definitely help you get those blissful ZZZs while you're still alive.

11 WHEN SLEEP GROWS ON TREES

This chapter is short and sweet... just like cherries.

Cherries, particularly Montmorency tart cherries,[xcv] are a particularly beneficial food source of melatonin that has been shown to improve sleep.[xcvi] I'm sure you've heard about melatonin before—our sleep hormone. Don't underestimate its power.

I have sometimes gone periods of time without taking tart cherry tablets at night, in order to save money. But I have needed to return to them to sleep better. Because I think I've insinuated that, as a former insomniac, I enjoy sleeping as well as possible.

I take two Cherry Works CherriMax tablets every night, and I'm not kidding when I say I can feel my melatonin kicking into high gear. Boost your melatonin from a food source where it is naturally occurring. Getting melatonin from cherries will help you sleep while you're still.

12 ABSORB YOUR NUTRIENTS

Up to this point we have looked at five very basic nutritional actions you can take to sleep well at night. 1. Avoiding Frankenfoods (okay, that's a *non*-action). 2. Drinking green smoothies. 3. Taking multivitamins. 4. Getting the sunshine vitamin. 5. Taking all-natural melatonin in the form of tart cherry supplements. This chapter is about something related but a little bit different—probiotics.

This book is all about nutrients, so you can imagine how important it is to *absorb* them!

This is where probiotics come in. I'm sure you've heard of them. They are live organisms that Dr. Johnson calls "friendly" or "good" bacteria that help us absorb certain nutrients.[xcvii] Probiotics have a profound effect on our gut, [xcviii] [xcix] where up to 80% of our immune system is located![c] Yet another benefit of probiotics is increased sleep![ci]

You can take probiotic supplements, and you can eat and drink them naturally in fermented foods and beverages. For a great-tasting beverage, try kombucha, which is fermented tea.

I took Vitacost Probiotic 15-35 15 Strains -- 35 billion CFU every day for a few years. They got my digestive health into really good shape, so I usually don't feel a need to take them anymore. (Warning: I felt sick the first few weeks I took them, as the bad bacteria was dying off, and then I felt great!) I have also really enjoyed kombucha on many occasions.

Probiotics helped my gut health a lot, and I feel like my nutrients are being well absorbed now. I recommend using probiotics for *at least* one long period in your life—they just might help you sleep while you're still alive.

13 I KNOW THIS SOUNDS CRAZY

I have a strange-sounding suggestion, but don't throw this book across the room (for the third time). We're getting so close to the end!

Every day, for as often as you are willing, put a teaspoon or two of organic virgin coconut oil in your mouth and swish it around *for at least 20 minutes*. Then spit it out in the trash or ground outside, rinse your mouth, floss, and brush. After a little while, "oil pulling", as it's called, can be done less frequently or when sleep is suffering.

You thought this book wasn't *too* crazy...until now. But I recommend oil pulling because it makes me feel like I pass out cold when my head hits the pillow. (As a former insomniac, I love sleeping like I'm in a coma).

I'm not the only one who feels that way. Oil pulling has been used in traditional medicine to help insomnia.[cii] Dr. F. Karach claimed sleeplessness is cured by oil pulling.[ciii] But why?

I'm not sure we know. What we *do* know from scientific studies is that oil pulling removes bacteria from the mouth. [civ][cv][cvi][cvii][cviii][cix]

Dentist Jessica T. Emery says bacteria hiding in the mouth's crevices are pulled out by oil pulling.[cx] She says many diseases and conditions are affected by the mouth's bacteria.[cxi] Jon Barron explains that harmful bacteria that form plaque get absorbed into the bloodstream from the mouth, but oil pulling stops these toxins from entering the body.[cxii]

I had to include oil pulling because of the difference I notice in my sleep. I used to practice it daily and now only need to occasionally, sometimes weekly. This may just be the strangest sounding thing you've never hear of, but don't risk not trying it. It might help you sleep while you're still alive.

14 WHAT I DO EVERY DAY

You stayed with me all through my recommendations. Thank you so much. That means that if you threw this book across the room, you picked it back up again. I'm so glad you did.

I have told you the nutritional actions I take personally, and I'm going to tell you again in this nice, neat bullet list below, because these things *just might* help you as much as they help me!

I avoid Frankenfoods. I eat whole foods with as few food additives as possible. Some food additives (especially excitotoxins) I avoid with a ten-foot pole.

Every morning, I take the following:

- *Vitamin B-6, B-12 & Folate* made by Food Research (one capsule).

- *Zhou Nutrition K2 + D3* (one capsule, which contains 5,000 IUs of D3). In the winter, I add an additional 10,000 IU of Vitamin D3 made by Healthy Origins (one softgel).

- *Vitamin-Mineral* made by Food Research (two tablets).

In either the afternoon or the evening, I make a green smoothie.

Then, about half an hour before bedtime, I take:

- CherriMax Tart Cherry Tablets made by Cherry Works (2 tablets).

Things I've done but don't do daily:

- Every day for about three years, I took Vitacost Probiotic 15-35 15 Strains -- 35 billion CFU. I still take these sometimes.

- I practiced oil pulling daily for a couple of weeks. I now practice it anywhere from occasionally to a few times a week.

Before we say goodbye, I have just a little more encouragement for you.

Are there stressful obligations, relationships, or other circumstances you can remove from your life? Would a lifestyle change reduce your stress? Several years ago, I pursued working and living in a small town with a slow pace of life and no work commute. This greatly increased my quality of life and my down time. I have also removed obligations and even relationships that had taken a toll on my mental health. Maybe you can, too. In addition, a spiritual worldview and spiritual activities such as prayer and church services are a huge help to me in providing the kind of comfort that lends itself to sleeping well.

Even as you practice the things in this book, don't "try" to sleep. Trying to sleep puts pressure on yourself, which isn't sleep-inducing. Just get the right stuff in your body and go on with your life. Cross things off your to-do list. Journal about what's bothering you. Seek a peaceful life, inwardly and outwardly. Cry when you need to; it can help reduce your stress.[cxiii]

This book stems from my heartfelt desire for you to sleep better. It's based on my real day-to-day life. I'm prone to insomnia and have been through the worst of it, yet I sleep well as long as I follow my own recommendations in this book. I hope you will give all of them a chance.

I will end with a reminder about my car analogy. I like that analogy a lot and can't get enough of it. So here goes again. Putting gas in a car is totally necessary to make it run. No matter what else might be wrong with the car, you'd always make sure it had fuel. Similarly, getting the right stuff in your body is foundational to sleeping well. If you want to look for other causes and cures for insomnia, you can; but always make sure you've got the basics covered first. What I mean is, if you are getting enough nutrients, then other supplements could begin to help. For example, I now take molecular hydrogen tablets each night and find myself sleeping deeper and remembering my dreams more often. I don't consider these essential, but I do consider them helpful. There are all kinds of supplements that may make you feel better and sleep better if you first have a proper nutritional foundation. If you do, you may just sleep while you're still alive.

WILL YOU RATE MY BOOK?

Sleep While You're Still Alive is self-published. If you believe my book can help others, please consider rating and reviewing it on Amazon. As a self-published author, the only ones getting my book out there are me and possibly you. Ratings and reviews make my book much more likely to be noticed. Thank you! -Audrey

ABOUT THE AUTHOR

Audrey Wagner is the author of *Klonopin Withdrawal and Howling Dogs* and *Divorcing Facebook? Really!?* She has an undergraduate degree in Philosophy and graduate degrees in Counseling and Theological Studies. She enjoys reading, writing, photography, nature, church, and time with family and friends. You can visit Audrey at her Amazon Author Page.

ENDNOTES

[i] S. Schutte-Rodin et al., "Clinical Guideline for the Evaluation and Management of Chronic Insomnia in Adults," *Journal of Clinical Sleep Medicine* 4, no.5, (October 2008): 487-504, https://www.ncbi.nlm.nih.gov/pubmed/18853708.

[ii] Schutte-Rodin et al., "Clinical Guideline."

[iii] Abigail Zuger, "Is Insomnia A Disease?" *Medscape*, accessed April 03, 2017, https://www.medscape.com/viewarticle/749277_1.

[iv] "Treatment," Insomnia, National Sleep Foundation, accessed March 21, 2017, https://sleepfoundation.org/insomnia/content/treatment.

[v] "Prescription sleeping pills: What's right for you?" Mayo Clinic, December 27, 2014, http://www.mayoclinic.org/diseases-conditions/insomnia/in-depth/sleeping-pills/art-20043959.

[vi] "How Is Insomnia Treated?" National Heart Lung and Blood Institute, last modified December 13, 2011, https://www.nhlbi.nih.gov/health/health-topics/topics/inso/treatment.

[vii] Michel Billiard and Alison Bentley, "Is Insomnia Best Categorized as a Symptom or a Disease?" *Sleep Medicine* 5, no. 1 (June 2004): S35-S40, https://doi.org/10.1016/S1389-9457(04)90006-8.

[viii] "Insomnia," Mayo Clinic, October 15, 2016, http://www.mayoclinic.org/diseases conditions/insomnia/symptoms-causes/syc-20355167.

[ix] Veronique Greenwood, "Pharma Watch: A User's Guide to Sleeping Pills," *Scientific American*, last modified January 01, 2016, https://www.scientificamerican.com/article/pharma-watch-a-user-s-guide-to-sleeping-pills/.

[x] Michael J. Sateia et al., "Clinical Practice Guideline for the Pharmacologic Treatment of Chronic Insomnia in Adults: An American Academy of Sleep Medicine Clinical Practice Guideline," *Journal of Clinical Sleep Medicine* 13, no. 2 (February 2017): 307-49, http://doi.org/10.5664/jcsm.6470

[xi] Sateia et al., "Clinical Practice Guideline."

[xii] Sateia et al., "Clinical Practice Guideline."

[xiii] Daniel F. Kripke, "Hypnotic Drug Risks of Mortality, Infection, Depression, and Cancer: But Lack of Benefit," *F1000Research* 5, no. 918 (May 2016), http://doi.org/10.12688/f1000research.8729.1.

[xiv] Sateia et al., "Clinical Practice Guideline."

[xv] Sateia et al., "Clinical Practice Guideline."

[xvi] Kripke, "Hypnotic Drug Risks."

[xvii] Sateia et al., "Clinical Practice Guideline."

[xviii] Sateia et al., "Clinical Practice Guideline."

[xix] Tais Araujo et al., "Qualitative Studies of Insomnia: Current State of Knowledge in the Field, " *Sleep Medicine Reviews* 31 (February 2017): 58-69, http://doi.org/10.1016/j.smrv.2016.01.003.

[xx] S. Schutte-Rodin et al., "Clinical Guideline for the Evaluation and Management of Chronic Insomnia in Adults," *Journal of Clinical Sleep Medicine* 4, no.5, (October 2008): 487-504, https://www.ncbi.nlm.nih.gov/pubmed/18853708.

[xxi] Jeanne M. Geiger-Brown et al., "Cognitive Behavioral Therapy in Persons with Comorbid Insomnia: A Meta-analysis," *Sleep Medicine Reviews* 23 (October 2015): 54-67, http://doi.org/10.1016/j.smrv.2014.11.007.

[xxii] James M. Trauer et al., "Cognitive Behavioral Therapy for Chronic Insomnia: A Systematic Review and Meta-analysis," *Annals of Internal Medicine* 163, no. 3 (August 2015): 191-204, http://doi.org/10.7326/m14-2841.

[xxiii] Charles M. Morin and Ruth M. Benca, "Nature, Evaluation, and Treatment of Insomnia," *Sleep Disorders Medicine* (May 2017): 673-696, http://doi.org/10.1007/978-1-4939-6578-6_37.

[xxiv] Dallas Hartwig and Melissa Hartwig, *It Starts with Food* (Las Vegas: Victory Belt Publishing, 2014), 76.

[xxv] Russell Blaylock, "Inflammation Causes Insomnia," *Newsmax*, February 23, 2017, http://www.newsmax.com/Health/Dr-Blaylock/inflammation-insomnia-melatonin-hesperidin/2017/02/23/id/775181/.

[xxvi] Jihui Zhang et al., "Differentiating Nonrestorative Sleep

from Nocturnal Insomnia Symptoms: Demographic, Clinical, Inflammatory, and Functional Correlates," *Sleep* 36, no. 5 (May 2013): 671-79, http://doi.org/10.5665/sleep.2624.

[xxvii] Michael R. Irwin, Richard Olmstead, and Judith E. Carroll, "Sleep Disturbance, Sleep Duration, and Inflammation: A Systematic Review and Meta-Analysis of Cohort Studies and Experimental Sleep Deprivation," *Biological Psychiatry* 80, no. 1 (July 2016): 40-52, http://doi.org/10.1016/j.biopsych.2015.05.014.

[xxviii] Hyong Jin Cho et al., "Sleep Disturbance and Longitudinal Risk of Inflammation: Moderating Influences of Social Integration and Social Isolation in the Coronary Artery Risk Development in Young Adults (CARDIA) Study," *Brain, Behavior, and Immunity* 46 (May 2015): 319-26. http://doi.org/10.1016/j.bbi.2015.02.023.

[xxix] Maria Basta et al., "Chronic Insomnia and the Stress System," *Sleep Medicine Clinics* 2, no. 2 (June 2007): 279-91, http://doi.org/10.1016/j.jsmc.2007.04.002.

[xxx]David R. Seaman, *The Deflame Diet: Deflame Your Diet, Body, and Mind* (Wilmington, NC: Shadow Panther Press, 2016), 23, Kindle.

[xxxi] Don Colbert, *What Would Jesus Eat?* (Nashville: Thomas Nelson, Inc., 2002), chap. 1, Kindle.

[xxxii] Sara Sarrafi Zadeh and Khyrunnisa Begum, "Comparison of Nutrient Intake by Sleep Status in Selected Adults in Mysore, India," *Nutrition Research and Practice* 5, no. 3 (June 2011): 230-35, http://doi.org/10.4162/nrp.2011.5.3.230.

[xxxiii] Mei-Yen Chen, Edward K. Wang, and Yi-Jong Jeng, "Adquate Sleep among Adolescents Is Positively Associated with Health Status and Health-related Behaviors," *BMC Public Health* 6, no. 59 (March 2006), http://doi.org/10.1186/1471-2458-6-59.

[xxxiv] Basta et al., "Chronic Insomnia and the Stress System."

[xxxv] Vicki B. Griffin, Edwin Neblett, and Evelyn Kissinger, "Stress Effects on Nutrition," *Lifestyle Laboratory*, accessed December 5, 2017, http://lifestylelaboratory.com/articles/stress-effects-nutrition.html.

[xxxvi] Emily J. Watson et al., "Caffeine Consumption and Sleep Quality in Australian Adults," *Nutrients* 8, no. 8 (August 2016): 479, http://doi.org/10.3390/nu8080479.

[xxxvii] Ian Clark and Hans Peter Landolt, "Coffee, Caffeine, and Sleep: A Systematic Review of Epidemiological Studies and Randomized Controlled Trials," *Sleep Medicine Reviews* 31 (February 2017): 70-78, http://doi.org/10.1016/j.smrv.2016.01.006.

[xxxviii] Sam Robbins, "Top 10 Caffeine Related Health Problems," *HFL Solutions*, accessed April 25, 2017, https://www.hflsolutions.com/ne/free_articles/CaffeineProblems_Top10.pdf.

[xxxix] Clark and Landolt, "Coffee, Caffeine, and Sleep."

[xl] Robbins, "Top 10 Caffeine Related Health Problems."

[xli] Institute of Medicine (US) Food Forum, "Nutrition Concerns for Aging Populations," in *Providing Healthy and Safe Foods As We Age: Workshop Summary*, (January 2010), https://www.ncbi.nlm.nih.gov/books/NBK51837/.

[xlii] Mariangela Rondanelli et al., "The Effect of Melatonin, Magnesium, and Zinc on Primary Insomnia in Long-Term Care Facility Residents in Italy: A Double-Blind, Placebo-Controlled Clinical Trial," *Journal of the American Geriatrics Society* 59, no. 1 (January 2011): 82-90, http://doi.org/10.1111/j.1532-5415.2010.03232.x.

[xliii] Natsuko Sato-Mito et al., "The Midpoint of Sleep Is Associated with Dietary Intake and Dietary Behavior among Young Japanese Women," *Sleep Medicine* 12, no. 3 (March 2011): 289-94, http://doi.org/10.1016/j.sleep.2010.09.012.

[xliv] Michael A. Grandner et al., "Sleep Symptoms Associated with Intake of Specific Dietary Nutrients," *Journal of Sleep Research* 23, no. 1 (February 2014): 22-34, http://doi.org/10.1111/jsr.12084.

[xlv] Xiao Tan et al., "Effect of Six-Month Diet Intervention on Sleep among Overweight and Obese Men with Chronic Insomnia Symptoms: A Randomized Controlled Trial," *Nutrients* 8, no. 11 (November 2016): 751, http://doi.org/10.3390/nu8110751.

[xlvi] Xiao Tan et al., "Effect of Six-Month Diet Intervention on

Sleep among Overweight and Obese Men with Chronic Insomnia Symptoms: A Randomized Controlled Trial," *Nutrients* 8, no. 11 (November 2016): 751, http://doi.org/10.3390/nu8110751.

[xlvii] B. Abbasi and S. M. Kimigar, "The Effect of Magnesium Supplementation on Primary Insomnia in Elderly: A Double-Blind Placebo-Controlled Clinical Trial," *Nutrition and Food Sciences Research* 1, no. 1 (November-December 2014): 79, http://en.journals.sid.ir/ViewPaper.aspx?ID=433098.

[xlviii] Hsiao-Han Lin et al., "Effect of Kiwifruit Consumption on Sleep Quality in Adults with Sleep Problems," *Asia Pacific Journal of Clinical Nutrition* 20, no. 2 (2011): 169-74, https://www.ncbi.nlm.nih.gov/pubmed/21669584.

[xlix] Arden B. Andersen, *Real Medicine, Real Health* (Waynesville, NC: Holographic Health Press, 2004), 23.

[l] Mercola, Joseph. "Top 33 Tips to Optimize Your Sleep Routine." *Mercola*, 3 Jan. 2019, articles.mercola.com/sites/articles/archive/2019/01/03/tips-to-a-good-night-sleep.aspx.

[li] Kresser, Chris. "Not Eating Enough - 8 Signs That Show You Are Under-Eating." *Chris Kresser*, 19 June 2019, chriskresser.com/are-you-an-under-eater-8-signs-youre-not-eating-enough/.

[lii] Michael Pollan, *In Defense of Food: An Eater's Manifesto* (Saint Louis, MO: Turtleback Books, 2009), 11.

[liii] "Substances Added to Food (formerly EAFUS)," *U.S. Food & Drug Administration*, last modified April 22, 2019, https://www.accessdata.fda.gov/scripts/fdcc/?set=FoodSubstances.

[liv] Saly Fallon and Mary G. Enig, "The Skinny on Fats," *The Weston A. Price Foundation*, January 1, 2000, https://www.westonaprice.org/health-topics/know-your-fats/the-skinny-on-fats/#hd.

[lv] Fallon and Enig, "The Skinny of Fats."

[lvi] "How Excitotoxins like MSG Give You Insomnia," *Scientific Health*, September 11, 2012, http://www.scientifichealth.org/91/how-excitotoxins-like-msg-give-you-insomnia/.

[lvii] Zumin Shi et al., "Association between Monosodium Glutamate Intake and Sleep-disordered Breathing among Chinese Adults with Normal Body Weight," *Nutrition* 29, no. 3 (March 2013): 508-13, http://doi.org/10.1016/j.nut.2012.08.011.

[lviii] Victoria Boutenko, *Green for Life* (Berkeley, CA: North Atlantic Books, 2010), 10, 39.

[lix] Boutenko, *Green for Life*, 39-40.

[lx] Boutenko, *Green for Life*, 20-21.

[lxi] Boutenko, *Green for Life*, 135-158.

[lxii] Michael J. Breus, "Cooking up a Sleep-friendly Diet," *The Sleep Doctor*, August 6, 2012, https://www.thesleepdoctor.com/2012/08/06/cooking-up-a-sleep-friendly-diet/.

[lxiii] John B. Marler, and Jeanne R. Wallin, "Human Health, the Nutritional Quality of Harvested Food and Sustainable Farming Systems," *Nutrition Security Institute*, accessed March 21, 2017, http://nutritionsecurity.org/PDF/NSI_White%20Paper_Web.pdf.

[lxiv] "Insomnia: Studies Suggest Calcium And Magnesium Effective," *Medical News Today*, September 8, 2009, http://www.medicalnewstoday.com/releases/163169.php.

[lxv] Joseph Mercola, "Tips for Resetting Your Internal Clock and Sleeping Better," *Mercola*, August 15, 2013, https://articles.mercola.com/sites/articles/archive/2013/08/15/nutrients-better-sleep.aspx.

[lxvi] "Insomnia," *Medical News Today*.

[lxvii] Mercola, "Tips for Resetting."

[lxviii] "Magnesium," *The World's Healthiest Foods*, accessed March 21, 2017, http://www.whfoods.com/genpage.php?tname=nutrient&dbid=75.

[lxix] "Calcium," *The World's Healthiest Foods*, accessed March 21, 2017, http://www.whfoods.com/genpage.php?tname=nutrient&dbid=45#foodchart.

[lxx] "Potassium," *The World's Healthiest Foods*, accessed March

21, 2017,
http://www.whfoods.com/genpage.php?dbid=90&tname=nutrie
nt.

[lxxi] Boutenko, *Green for Life*, 101-103.
[lxxii] Christopher Masterjohn, "Nutritional Adjuncts to the Fat-Soluble Vitamins," *The Weston A. Price Foundation*, January 28, 2013, https://www.westonaprice.org/health-topics/abcs-of-nutrition/nutritional-adjuncts-to-the-fat-soluble-vitamins/.

[lxxiii] "Should you get your nutrients from food or from supplements? *Harvard Health Publishing*, May 2015, https://www.health.harvard.edu/staying-healthy/should-you-get-your-nutrients-from-food-or-from-supplements.
[lxxiv] Scott A. Johnson, *The Doctor's Guide to Surviving When Modern Medicine Fails: The Ultimate Natural Medicine Guide to Preventing Disease and Living Longer* (New York: Skyhorse Publishing, 2015), chap. 1, Kindle.
[lxxv] Marler and Wallin, "Human Health."
[lxxvi] Johnson, *The Doctor's Guide*, chap. 3.
[lxxvii] Johnson, *The Doctor's Guide*, chap. 3.
[lxxviii] Brian Clement, "Nutri-Con: The Truth About Vitamins & Supplements," *Organic Consumers Association*, December 31, 2006, https://www.organicconsumers.org/news/nutri-con-truth-about-vitamins-supplements.
[lxxix] Colleen Huber, "What to Look for in a Vitamin," *The American Association of Naturopathic Physicians*, accessed July 21, 2017, http://www.naturopathic.org/content.asp?contentid=35.

[lxxx] Robert Thiel, "The Truth About Vitamins in Nutritional Supplements," *Doctor's Research*, accessed July 26, 2017. http://www.doctorsresearch.com/articles4.html.
[lxxxi] Thiel, "The Truth About Vitamins."

[lxxxii] Thiel, "The Truth About Vitamins."
[lxxxiii] Thiel, "The Truth About Vitamins."
[lxxxiv] Joseph Mercola, "The World's Single Deadliest Vitamin Deficiency," *Mercola*, accessed March 21, 2017,

http://www.mercola.com/Downloads/bonus/vitamin-d/report.aspx

[lxxxv] Joseph Mercola, "Vitamin D—One of the Simplest Solutions to Wide-Ranging Health Problems," *Mercola*, December 22, 2013, https://articles.mercola.com/sites/articles/archive/2013/12/22/dr-holick-vitamin-d-benefits.aspx.

[lxxxvi] Christopher Masterjohn, "From Seafood to Sunshine: A New Understanding of Vitamin D Safety," *The Weston A. Price Foundation*, December 17, 2006, https://www.westonaprice.org/health-topics/abcs-of-nutrition/from-seafood-to-sunshine-a-new-understanding-of-vitamin-d-safety/.

[lxxxvii] Saly Fallon and Mary G. Enig, "Cod Liver Oil Basics and Recommendations," *The Weston A. Price Foundation*, February 9, 2009, https://www.westonaprice.org/health-topics/cod-liver-oil/cod-liver-oil-basics-and-recommendations/.

[lxxxviii] Michael J. Breus, "Low on Vitamin D, Sleep Suffers," *Huffpost*, last modified March 4, 2017, http://www.huffingtonpost.com/dr-michael-j-breus/low-on-vitamin-d-sleep-suffers_b_9332008.html.

[lxxxix] Jennifer Massa et al., "Vitamin D and Actigraphic Sleep Outcomes in Older Community-Dwelling Men: The MrOS Sleep Study," *Sleep* 38, no. 2 (February 2015): 251-57, http://doi.org/10.5665/sleep.4408.

[xc] Paul J. Veugelers and John Paul Edwaru, "A Statistical Error in the Estimation of the Recommended Dietary Allowance for Vitamin D," *Nutrients* 6, no. 10 (October 2014): 4472-75, http://doi.org/10.3390/nu6104472.

[xci] Mercola, "Vitamin D—One of the Simplest Solutions."

[xcii] Breus, "Low on Vitamin D."

[xciii] "How Do I Get the Vitamin D My Body Needs?" Vitamin D Council, accessed March 29, 2017, https://www.vitamindcouncil.org/about-vitamin-d/how-do-i-get-the-vitamin-d-my-body-needs/.

[xciv] "Testing for Vitamin D," *Vitamin D Council*, accessed

March 21, 2017, https://www.vitamindcouncil.org/testkit/.

[xcv] "Healthy Cherries," King Orchards, accessed September 19, 2017, https://kingorchards.com/healthy-cherries/.

[xcvi] Howatson, Glyn, et al. "Effect of Tart Cherry Juice (Prunus Cerasus) on Melatonin Levels and Enhanced Sleep Quality." *European Journal of Nutrition* 51, no. 8 (2011): 909–916, http://doi.org/10.1007/s00394-011-0263-7.

[xcvii] Johnson, *The Doctor's Guide*, chap. 3.

[xcviii] M. Choct, "Managing Gut Health through Nutrition," *British Poultry Science* 50, no. 1 (February 2009): 9-15, http://doi.org/10.1080/00071660802538632.

[xcix] C. Pagnini et al., "Probiotics Promote Gut Health through Stimulation of Epithelial Innate Immunity," *Proceedings of the National Academy of Sciences* 107, no. 1 (January 2010): 454-59, http://doi.org/10.1073/pnas.0910307107.

[c] Johnson, *The Doctor's Guide*, chap. 3.

[ci] "The Many Benefits Of Probiotics," Probiotics.org, accessed March 21, 2017, https://probiotics.org/benefits/.

[cii] "Oil Pulling: Safe, Simple and Effective!" *Earth Clinic*, November 4, 2017, http://www.earthclinic.com/remedies/oil_pulling.html.

[ciii] "Pulling Oil (The Oil Treatment of Dr. Karach)," *Oil Pulling—Wonderful Therapy*, accessed April 6, 2017, http://www.oilpulling.org/wp-content/uploads/2009/09/Pulling_Oil_Karach_Article.pdf.

[civ] T. Durai Anand et al., "Effect of Oil-pulling on Dental Caries Causing Bacteria," *African Journal of Microbiology* 2 (March 2008): 63-66, http://doi.org/10.5897/ajmr.

[cv] S. Asokan et al., "Effect of Oil Pulling on Streptococcus Mutanscount in Plaque and Saliva Using Dentocult SM Strip Mutans Test: A Randomized, Controlled, Triple-blind Study," *Journal of Indian Society of Pedodontics and Preventive Dentistry* 26, no. 1 (March 2008): 12-17, http://doi.org/10.4103/0970-4388.40315.

[cvi] Poonam Sood, et al., "Comparative Efficacy of Oil Pulling and Chlorhexidine on Oral Malodor : A Randomized Controlled

Trial," *Journal Of Clinical And Diagnostic Research* 8, no. 11
(November 2014): 18-21,
http://doi.org/10.7860/jcdr/2014/9393.5112.

[cvii] Faizalc Peedikayil, Prathima Sreenivasan, and Arun
Narayanan, "Effect of Coconut Oil in Plaque Related Gingivitis - A
Preliminary Report," *Nigerian Medical Journal* 56, no. 2
(March/April 2015): 143-47, http://doi.org/10.4103/0300-
1652.153406.

[cviii] Mamta Kaushik et al., "The Effect of Coconut Oil Pulling
on Streptococcus Mutans Count in Saliva in Comparison with
Chlorhexidine Mouthwash," *The Journal of Contemporary Dental
Practice* 17, no. 1 (January 2016): 38-41, http://doi.org/10.5005/jp-
journals-10024-1800.

[cix] L.A. Sechi et al., "Antibacterial Activity of Ozonized
Sunflower Oil (Oleozon)," *Journal of Applied Microbiology* 90, no. 2
(February 2001): 279-84, http://doi.org/10.1046/j.1365-
2672.2001.01235.x.

[cx] Jessica T. Emery, "How Dental Professionals Can Respond
to 'oil Pulling' Patients," *DentistryiQ*, March 21, 2014,
http://www.dentistryiq.com/articles/2014/03/how-dental-
professionals-can-respond-to-oil-pulling-patients.html.

[cxi] Emery, "How Dental Professionals."

[cxii] Jon Barron. "Oil Pulling For Detoxing? No, But Helps With
Gum Disease & Immunity -- Natural Health Newsletter," *Baseline
of Health Foundation*, April 4, 2011,
https://jonbarron.org/article/oil-pulling-detoxing.

[cxiii] Murube, Juan. "Hypotheses on the Development of
Psychoemotional Tearing." *The Ocular Surface*, vol. 7, no. 4, 2009,
pp. 171–175., doi:10.1016/s1542-0124(12)70184-2.

Made in the USA
Coppell, TX
21 January 2023

11468314R00056